Just meditate...
...could do you some good

Sandra Rauchenecker

Author: Sandra Rauchenecker

Cover design: Christian Rauchenecker
Design from Munich, www.rauchenecker.com

ISBN: 9781079278361

QUOTE

"**Meditation** is not about trying to get anywhere. It is about allowing ourselves to be exactly where we are, to be exactly as we are, and to allow the world to be exactly as it is at that moment."

Jon Kabat-Zinn

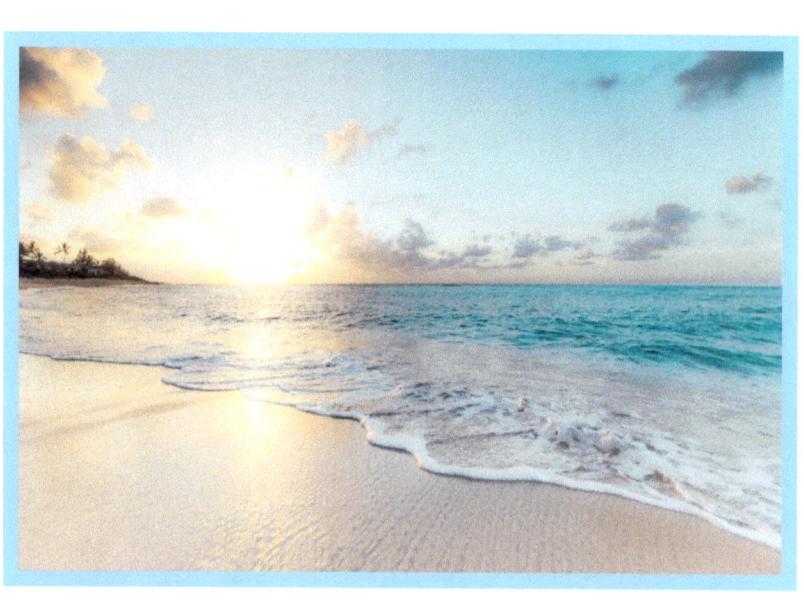

CONTENT

Content

Introduction

Perhaps you are familiar with this, everyday life with all kinds of appointments always has you firmly under control, you rush from one appointment to the next, always worried about coming late or forgetting something important. You are trapped in the hamster wheel of everyday life. No time to rest, take a deep breath, just let your soul dangle... The first symptoms quickly become noticeable: Sleeplessness, restlessness, heart palpitations, fluctuations in feelings.

Therefore meditation is one of the most important things we can learn for our life. Especially in today's world, where more and more people suffer from stress, insomnia, anxiety, overexertion, over-stimulation, it is important to know a simple but very effective method that helps you to get back to your center, helps you to sleep better again, to be healthier, to concentrate better. From a spiritual point of view, meditation is much more than just relaxation. It is about finding inner peace, detached from compulsions, but also wishes of the ego.

In fact, there are studies that show that if you allow yourself and your thoughts only a few minutes of meditation each day, your stress level will be significantly lowered and your quality of life increased. With the help of meditation you will improve your physical as well as your mental well-being. Both work hand in hand. In this book I would like to show you how you can change your life easily and quickly by meditating.

I will take you into a world whose advantages are still almost completely unknown to many people. Are you still skeptical? What is there to lose except a few minutes a day when you can at least try? I am sure that after one or two meditation exercises you will want to continue. There are many different ways to meditate, we look at the best and the simplest together.

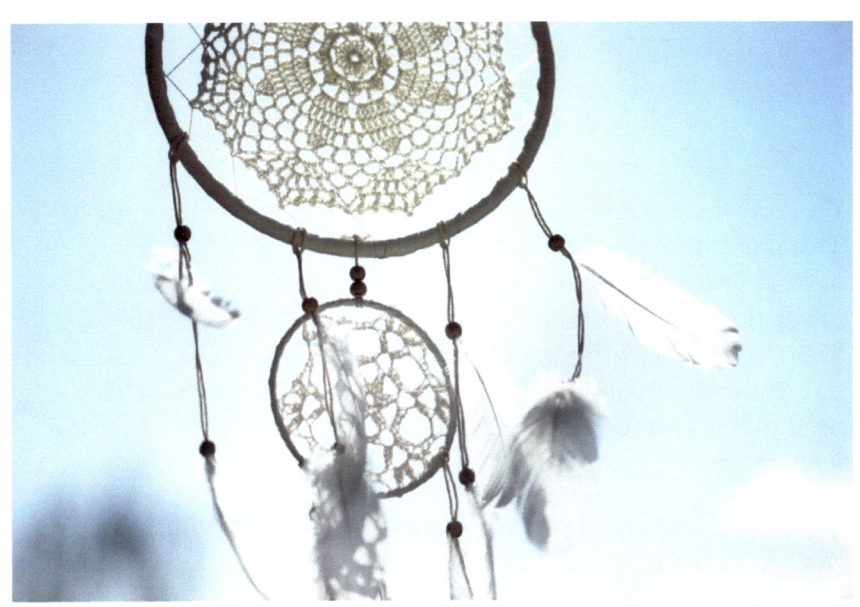

Meditation for beginners

We've all learned a lot and somewhere we had to start learning it. This is also true for meditation. There is nothing more beautiful than to be at peace with yourself. So get involved in the adventure of meditation with joy and ease. It will improve your life by 100%. These techniques for beginners will help you make wise decisions and direct your attention where you need it to be. To start with, all you need to do is just want it and get started. Just try it out and see if it does you good. Then you can still deepen the techniques.

There is no "right way" to do it! Don't worry about things like choosing the best place to sit, what position to use or what to wear. Just find the most comfortable, quiet place to sit - bed, sofa or chair.

In the beginning, two to five minutes is enough - you may think it is easy to get fully into meditation, but that's not it! During the first two weeks you should meditate only two to five minutes a day and then slowly increase it by one minute every few days until it is up to 10 minutes a day at the end of the month.

Turn meditation into a morning routine or evening routine - Simple, isn't it? So take your time, mark it in your calendar and meditate every morning or evening for two to five minutes.

Don't forget to pay attention to your feelings - watch how your body feels and how your mental state is (anxious, busy or tired). If you understand your feelings, accept them and be at peace with yourself during meditation.

Establish a loving attitude - Many thoughts and feelings will arise during meditation. Notice them without judging.

Count your breaths to 10 - Breathe in and out through your nose, trace the path of your breath. Count each breath, calm and relaxed. Count to 10. Start all over.

The mind will wander and that's fine - when this happens, just smile gently and return to counting. At first you may sometimes be frustrated. But everything is fine. Everything takes time.

You are not doing it wrong - don't worry about how you are doing it. There is no perfect way to do it. Find your own way.

Should you worry about freeing the mind? Focus on the exercise. When a thought arises, turn your attention back to your breathing. Over time, your thoughts will become less and less distracting.

Get to know yourself - meditation focuses your attention. Just observe the "activities" of your mind during meditation and you will be surprised how much you will learn about yourself.

Everywhere is the perfect place for meditation - whether in a bus, train, plane, a bank in a public park or at home, every place is a good place to meditate.

If you wish, you can also try guided meditation - many use guided meditation, so it's perfectly all right for you to try. But always alternate with meditations where you are in silence.

Your best friend is yourself - learn to appreciate yourself more, smile and give yourself love instead of criticism. Be your best friend. Start to perceive the light, the sounds and the energy around you. Perceive only the light around you on one day, the sounds on the other and the energy on another.

Smile after meditation - Be grateful for the time you have spent with yourself. In this way you show yourself worthy. I wish you a lot of joy with your first steps into your meditation practice and as always I am looking forward to hearing your feedback. And now we go a little deeper and expand your meditation practice, because now you are already an advanced.

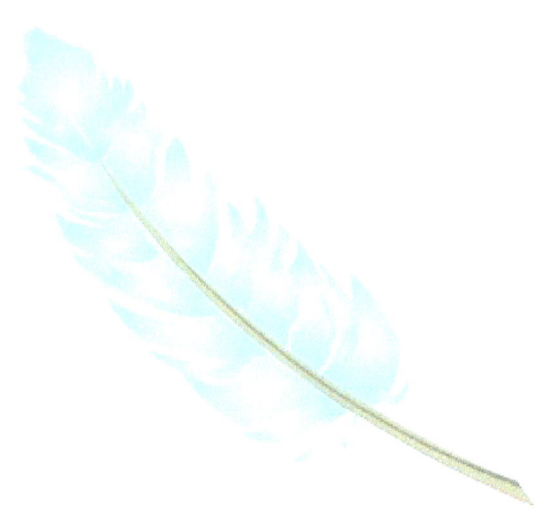

Whas is Meditation?

The term meditation is derived from the Latin word meditari which means to reflect, to think, and contemplate. Mediation is a spiritual practice practiced in many cultures. The mind should be calmed by mindfulness and/or concentration exercises.

Meditating means

To be simple, with no goal and no intention, without having to do anything

- Being in the here and now, quite present
- To observe the events, quietly, without judging, accepting what wishes to show itself
- To let the stream of thoughts come to rest
- To be mindful and conscious
- To perceive thoughts, feelings and sensations
- Allow silence and experience peace

How does meditation benefit you?

Meditation is the best way to bring your body, mind and soul into harmony. With regular practice you will become calmer, more relaxed, healthier, more concentrated, more mindful and more conscious. Meditation does not take you away from life, it helps you to live better. This is how meditation affects your life:

Physically

- Relief from chronic pain
- Strengthening of the immune system
- Stimulation of self-healing powers
- Too high blood pressure is lowered

- Better sleep
- Improved posture
- Better body awareness
- Better memory
- Weight control
- Can help release addiction in any form

Mental

- More balance
- More tolerance towards yourself and others
- More joy of life
- You feel (again) more gratitude
- You develop compassion for yourself and for others your self-love is encouraged.
- It contributes to personal and spiritual development
- Meditation is food for body, soul and spirit.

History of Meditation

Meditation is an art form that comes from all types of cultures and ancient civilizations. However, each form comes from a different place, which distinguishes it a little from the others. In India, for example, meditation was practiced several thousand years before Christ. Meditation was also known in ancient Egypt, as preserved wall reliefs show. Even in early Christianity as well as in Islam and Judaism different meditation techniques were used. Meditation originated in the East, from where it gradually spread across the Silk Road to us in the West. Starting from America, the practice of meditation gradually conquered Europe. Today, an increasing number of people are practicing meditation with us and are aware of its benefits for their own lives, and this trend will certainly continue to increase.

If you go a little deeper into the topic of meditation, you will find that meditation is practiced differently all over the world. You will find different names for different techniques and styles. In addition, you will find numerous religious and mystical additions. You will find many different things and many different approaches, depending on where the origin of the respective meditation technique lies. Ultimately, all techniques and styles aim at one and the same thing: To relax the body, mind and soul, to bring them into harmony and to experience silence. In the ancient Christian training of the mind, for example, meditation is the process of thinking, in which one deals with a topic with the highest concentration. In Eastern meditation, on the other hand, the aim of meditation is to detach oneself from everything, to distance oneself from thoughts and to experience silence. If you can do this, your mind will become very calm.

In the Eastern meditation arts this is called relaxation resonance, with which your body reacts. In the Christian, mystical exercises one speaks of contemplation.

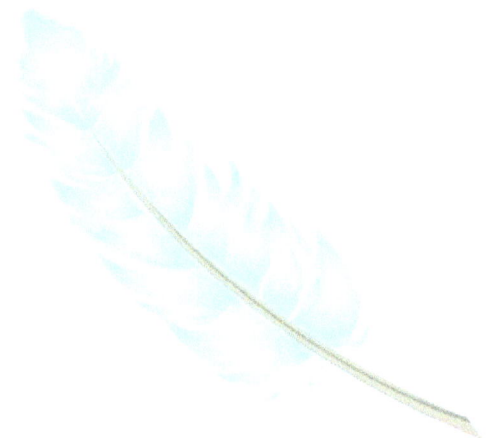

Preparations

Practice your breathing. Breathing means life. Your breath is the connection between your body and your soul. Observe your breath. How do you breathe? Deep into your stomach as it would be right to supply your body with oxygen? Or do you breathe shallowly and superficially? Breathing techniques are particularly suitable for relaxation and you can also use them without meditation for yourself and your well-being. If you are stressed or anxious, breathe flat into the upper chest area. This increases your pulse, your heart beats faster and your nervousness. If, on the other hand, you breathe slowly and take a deep breath, your heartbeat calms down and so does the thought carousel in your head. Why is that so? Body, soul and spirit are one, everything is connected. If you now change your stress symptoms on the physical level, e.g. through breathing exercises, this will also have an immediate effect on your soul and spirit. Breathing exercises are often combined with meditation. When you inhale and exhale, you concentrate only on the oxygen that flows in and out of your lungs and follow your breath with attention so that you don't think so much about other things. Breathing also helps you to relieve stress and anxiety and relax your body... It is especially important to train breathing at the beginning of the meditation practice. So take enough time, you will need it later for all other types of meditation..

Let's do a few breathing exercises right away

Deep abdominal breathing
- Sit up straight or lie on your back. Put one hand on the lower abdomen and breathe in deeply.
- Feel the air lifting your belly.
- Now try to breathe more slowly and evenly into the lower abdomen.
- The rhythm feels very natural.
- The breath flows and is not forced. Concentrate on this breathing as long as you like.

If you want to deepen your relaxation, close your eyes during this exercise

Ujjayi - Breathing technique

This technique allows you to focus and relax better. It is called "Sea Noise Breathing" because you can hear the sound of breathing in your throat.

- Sit up straight and imagine breathing on a mirror. This creates an "H" sound that sounds like the sound of the ocean in your throat. Now take a deep breath and try to create this H-noise while exhaling. Repeat breathing a few times.
- Now inhale, but then keep your mouth closed. You can now feel the "H" inside, the throat narrows slightly and the sound comes from the vocal chords.
- Repeat this a few times.
- You can now try out whether you can also generate the sound of the sea when you inhale.

Nadi shodana – Alternating breathing

- With the help of this breathing technique you harmonize the energies between the two halves of the brain.
- Sit up straight and breathe in and out slowly.
- Now close the right nostril with your thumb and breathe in very slowly and completely through the left nostril.
- At the end of inhalation, close both nostrils for one to two seconds.

- Now close the left nostril and exhale slowly and completely through the right nostril.
- Then hold your whole nose for a maximum of two seconds and hold your breath.

- Now close the left nostril, breathe in through the right, then stop breathing, keep the right nostril closed and breathe out through the left.

You can repeat this a few times

Test for yourself which breathing technique you can best cope with. You can also practice this at the bus stop or when you are standing in a traffic jam. The breathing techniques can also calm you down without meditation.

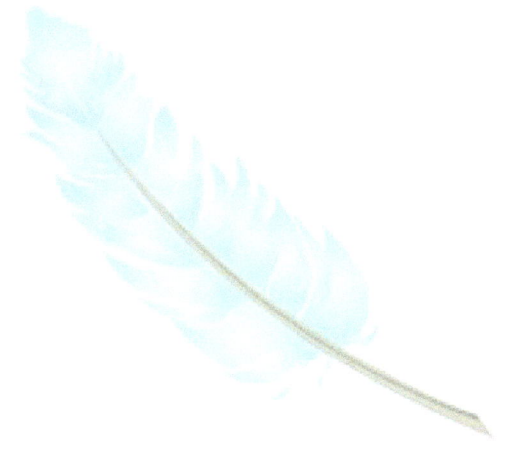

Create a beautiful atmosphere

The Room –- If you have already done a few meditation exercises and would like to meditate more often and regularly, you can now perhaps set up a meditation corner and even a meditation room. It would be best to meditate daily. But in everyday life it can happen that your wish fades again or you don't take the time. If you then have a beautifully designed meditation corner, it will remind you of your intention and you will be a little more excited to linger in such a beautiful place and come to rest. The environment you choose for meditation is one of the most important things to take care of. Find a quiet place where you can be alone and not disturbed. You should feel safe and secure there. If you can only use a small part of a room for meditation, then visually separate it from the rest of the room. You could set up a screen or hang a plant, a picture on the wall, a nice carpet on the floor. Make sure that all sources of interference, such as telephone, mobile phone are switched off and ask your family not to disturb you now. Air the room well before you start meditating, maybe you have a blanket ready, sometimes it can be cold and if you are cold, you can't meditate well. Warm socks can also be very useful. If you like, you can light a candle, put a crystal in front of you or a flower. Also an essential fragrance oil, if you like it, can help you to relax.

Time – Choose an appropriate time for you, this can be in the morning after getting up, or in the evening before going to sleep. It is good if you meditate at the same time every day, body and mind will get used to it faster. Start with a maximum of 5 minutes meditation time, which is sufficient for the beginning. You will be surprised how long 5 minutes can be if you sit still and do your exercise. To avoid constantly looking at your watch when the 5 minutes are up, it is helpful to set an alarm clock or timer that tells you when the meditation time is up. Because every time you would open your eyes to look at the clock, you would get out of the relaxation phase and move away from your focus. I recorded you a small audio file, at the beginning and at the end a bell sounds, in the 5 minutes in between there is silence. If you like, you can download this audio file as mp3 and download it to your iPod.

www.sandra-rauchenecker.com/downloads/meditation/5minuten.mp3

Sitting or lying? For starters I would recommend you to meditate while sitting. You can easily sit on a chair. Make sure your feet touch the floor and your spine is straight. Place your hands loosely on your thighs, palms up. You can sit on the floor, on a meditation cushion. Here the cross-legged or lotus position has proved its worth. Make sure you have a straight spine. The hands lie loosely on the thighs with the palms upwards. Of course you can also medidate while lying down, but there is the risk that you fall asleep quickly. Just try out for yourself which method is best for you and what you feel most comfortable with.

Prepare yourself

Before you start with your first exercise, here are a few tips on how best to prepare yourself:

-   – Wear comfortable clothes that don't limit your movement
-   – Do not meditate after a sumptuous meal
-   – Don't meditate when you're under time constraints.

Going to the bathroom first can be helpful.

Various forms of meditation

Meditation of Mindfulness - Mindfulness is a way to think only of the present moment and not be overwhelmed by thoughts of the past or future. Mental health is very important and mindfulness can be an enormous help. With mindfulness you focus only on the present, so that you do not ponder sadly or anxiously about past or future events. It is an excellent way to reduce stress and anxiety, but it can also be useful for many other aspects of your life, from weight loss to increasing your productivity at work. Today, mindfulness is combined with meditation.

Why is mindfulness so important? Regular training of mindfulness helps you to have a better memory, increases your ability to concentrate and you are more focused overall. The meditation of mindfulness is also very beneficial for your body. Studies have shown that your body can fight infections better because mindfulness meditation strengthens your immune system. Let's start by practicing mindfulness meditation. First of all, you have to understand that not everything is going to be perfect immediately. Practice makes perfect" also applies here. Just start, don't put yourself under pressure, and don't let yourself be stopped from trying again every day.

Concentrate on your breathing - As with any kind of meditation, at the beginning you focus only on your breathing. Breathe in and out. Every time you exhale, let go of your worries, fears and thoughts.

Think about your current condition - Take a moment now to think only about what is happening. Think about how you are right here and now and practice meditation. Don't think about yesterday or a month ago or a year ago. Don't think about what you will do next or what plans you have for the future. Just think of this moment here and now.

Imagine every single part of your body - If you have problems in clearing your mind and focusing only on the present, you can try to think about every part of your body. Concentrate and feel your fingers, arms, belly, back, shoulders, legs and toes. Listen to your heartbeat and concentrate on the air that flows in and out of your lungs.

Accept what happens - A large part of mindfulness is not only to be aware of the present, but also to accept it. No matter what happens, be ready to accept it and learn to appreciate it.

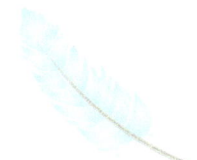

Meditation with a Mantra - A mantra is usually a short word or phrase that you say out loud or repeat in your mind and concentrate on to clear your mind. With a mantra you can also practice mindfulness again by concentrating on reciting the mantra and not on all the other thoughts and feelings that are so fond of buzzing around in your head. The more often you repeat your mantra, the more relaxed you become and the more you can clear your mind. For some people, complete silence makes their thoughts wander. If you repeat your mantra, it can also help you to reach a deeper/higher level of consciousness, which is also used in other types of meditation. Mantras are especially helpful for beginners as they calm the mind and prevent you from returning to all the other thoughts in your mind.

Choosing a Mantra - If you want to meditate with a mantra, it is important that you choose one that suits you, that you like, that is a positive, calming word, such as love or peace, before beginning your meditation. You should be able to remember it well and it should help you to think of nothing but this word, to come to rest and silence. The point is that you can relax and listen to the sound of your words. Let's take a look at some of the different mantras you could try. We will start with the old mantras that have been used for centuries:

OM (pronounced "AUM") - OM is a sacred syllable. One could

translate this mantra with "I am". This syllable symbolizes being and consciousness in any form. OM is the sacred sound of the universe, the "UR sound" so to speak. When you recite the OM during your meditation it harmonizes and centers you. Start with a meditation duration of 5 minutes.

Shanti - The syllable Shanti means peace and helps achieve inner balance, gives a feeling of happiness and harmony, liberates from fears and conflicts. If you carry peace within you, then you are capable of bonding and can connect with other people in a peaceful way. Peaceful people who rest within themselves are successful on both a private and professional level. Others like to be with such people. The peaceful, positive vibration transmits itself to others. If you like, practice meditation with the Mantra Shanti for a while. OM Shanti, Shanti, Shanti is interpreted in Hinduism as well as in Buddhism as triple peace in body, mind and soul.

OM Mani Padme Hum - is the mantra for compassion and healing. You can recite it during your meditation practice to express love and compassion - also and especially towards yourself - and thus find healing in this way. The Om Mani Padme Hum - Mantra empowers you to forgive yourself and others, the pain we have consciously or unconsciously caused. By reciting the mantra regularly, you assume the basic attitude of compassion. Instead of sinking into emotions like fear, despair, or anger, use the mantra, be mindful, and let every syllable become fully conscious, whether you speak it softly or loudly, or just think about it. But maybe you would rather use your own mantra, your own affirmation for your meditation practice. Then simply put together your own mantra. Depending on what is important and right for you and your current situation.

A couple of examples:

„My mind is clear"
„I am good as I am"
„I am in harmony with myself"
„ I am in the right place"

Or you recite individual words such as: peace - love - freedom - gratitude - harmony - oneness - light

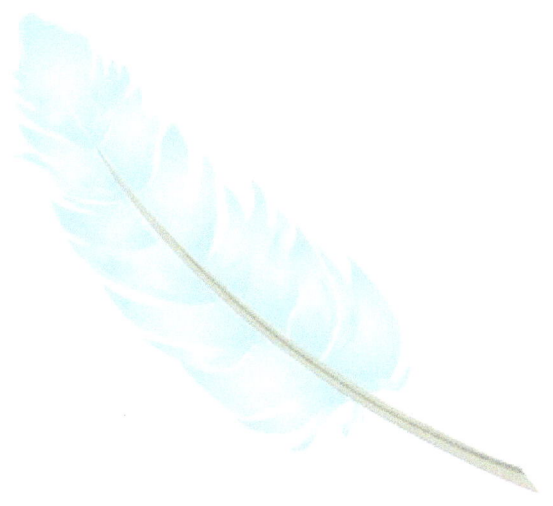

Chakra meditation. Chakras are energy centers in your body. Through these energy centers your body can send and receive energy. In order to meditate with the chakras, it is advantageous if you know where the chakras are. The 7 chakras are located in 7 different parts of your body.

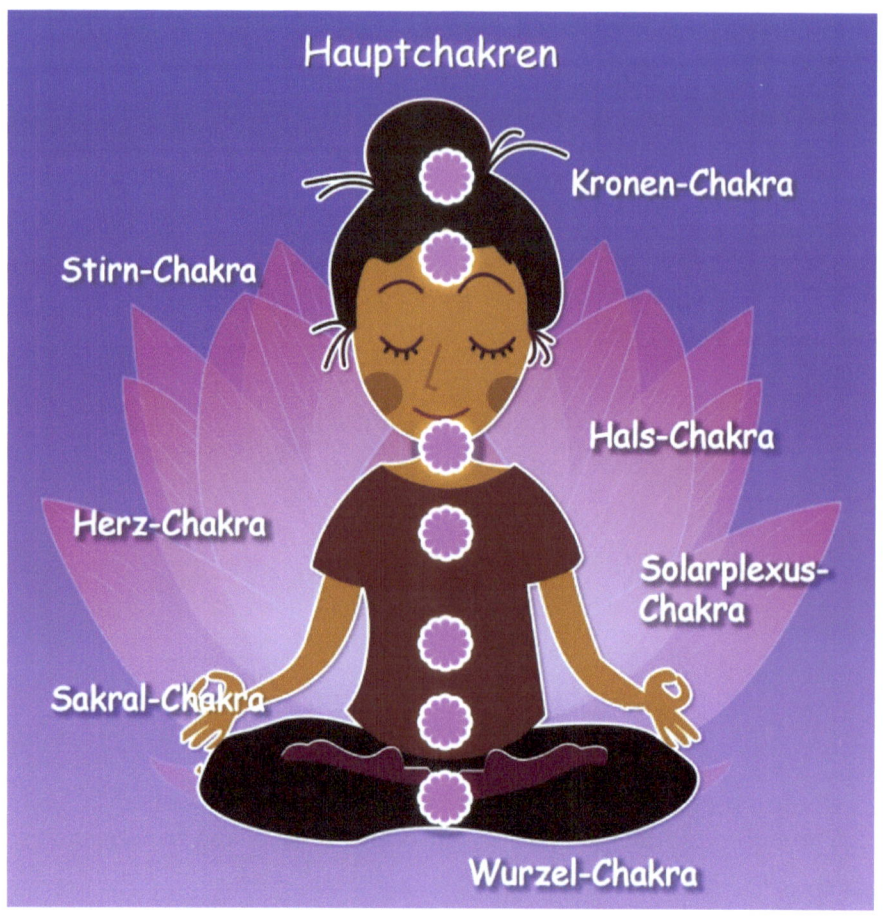

Root chakra - at the lower end of the spine * Sacral chakra - about a hand's width below the navel

* **Solar Plexus Chakra** - In the upper abdomen near the stomach
* **Heart chakra** - right above the heart and in the middle of the chest.
* **Neck chakra** - located in the neck, approximately at the larynx.
* **Forehead chakra** - in the middle of the forehead between the eyebrows
* **Crown chakra** - is located directly at the top of the crown and is referred to as the "crown

What does the chakras mean to you?

Root chakra – Your root chakra is located between the sacrum and coccyx, at the lower end of the spine between the hip bones. It is responsible for

- Your life force
- Your instincts
- Your safety
- Your survival
- Your material needs

Its color is RED. Function: connection to the earth, basic trust, stability, root for self-preservation, source of power for all activities, center of energy supply to the organism. The affirmation to open your root chakra is: "I am safe".

Sacral-Chakra – It is about 12 cm above your root chakra in the lumbar region, it is the chakra of emotion and creativity. It is responsible for

- Your creative power
- Your physical needs and preferences
- Your addictive behavior

It is the center of immediate, free flowing emotions, sensuality and sexual energy, distribution point of vital energies, seat of creative forces, enthusiasm and amazement. Its colour is ORANGE. The affirmation to open your sacral chakra is: "I am loved"

Solar plexus-Chakra – It is located in your stomach area and is important for your intuition, your gut feeling. It is responsible for

- Collective consciousness
- Power
- Control

Function: transformation of raw energy into subtle energy, processing of vital impulses, moods and feelings, activation of intellectual understanding, control of relationships and connections, seat of personal strength, self-confidence, development of contentment. The affirmation to open your solar plexus chakra is: "It is safe to know".

Heart-Chakra – It is located in the heart, in the middle of the chest. It is the chakra for

- Universal love
- Your complex emotions
- Your compassion
- Your love
- Your knowledge
- Your oneness and well-being

 Function: Source of healing, transformation of vital feelings into compassion and love, development of self-love and acceptance, development of the sense of beauty and harmony, control of emotions, regulation of the immune system. Its colours are LIGHT GREEN / PINK / SMARAGGREEN. Affirmation to open your heart chakra: "It is safe to love".

Neck chakra - It is located in the middle of the neck, it stands for

- Your wisdom
- Your communication
- Your growth
- Your manifestation
- Expressing your own truth

- Expressing your own truth
Function: connection of the physical and mental with the mental centers, distribution of creative energies, control of individual expression and communication, transformation of fear, emergence of joy, source of inner expanse, peace and inspiration His color is LIGHT BLUE. Affirmation for opening your laryngeal chakra: "It is safe to speak".

Forehead chakra. It is located between the eyes, a bit above the eyebrows. It is the energy center

- Your knowledge
- To your knowledge spiritual - emotional - physical
- Your consciousness
- Your clairvoyance
- Your intuition
- For the reception from "Above"

Function: Seat of intuitive and rational thinking as well as holistic insight, radiance and control of mental energies, manifestation through thought power, memory, visions and clairvoyance. Its color is DARK BLUE/INDIGOBLAUE Affirmation to open your forehead chakra: "It is safe to see".

Crown Chakra - It is located just above the center of your head, a bit above your body. It is the energy center

- Your consciousness
- Your bright knowledge
- Your divine guidance
- The direct line to "Top"
- Stands for cosmic consciousness
- Is the higher level of reality
- Pre-manifestation condition
- Premeditated creation
- Pure love and mercy

Function: opening man to the cosmos, experiencing the spiritual world, becoming aware of the All-Unity, devotion, union, perfection His colour is VIOLET/royal PURPLE. Affirmation for opening the crown chakra: "I know. I am aware. I love myself."

Now begin with your meditation

Sit or lie down, start concentrating on your breathing and then focus on one chakra at a time or on just one chakra every day... Imagine its colour as you concentrate on the chakra you want to work with today while at the same time paying attention to your breathing. Imagine that color - and breathing out. You can also concentrate on the corresponding physical organ, let's take the heart chakra as an example. Concentrate on your heart, feel your heartbeat, fill your chest with the green and pink colors, send love and compassion into your heart region. How does it feel? If you should concentrate on organs, please always imagine them healthy. You are also welcome to take the appropriate affirmation with you.

Guided meditation - Especially when you start meditating, it can be difficult to sit still and meditate alone. A guided meditation can help you. Here you will be guided through the meditation with a quiet, calming voice. Instructions are given on how to relax your body and purify your mind, different images help you to concentrate so that you can really relax.

Walk Meditation - Meditation does not always have to take place in a quiet, dark room where you have no distractions. Sometimes this exercise can also be done during other activities, such as walking. Let's talk about some things you should know about meditating while walking.

Why should you meditate while walking?

When you are walking, it is actually the perfect time to meditate. While walking, not only do you spend time alone with yourself, but you also focus more on the activity and the fresh air. You can concentrate a little better, but not in a way that makes you think about stressful things. It is a way to concentrate on nothing and just clear the mind. You can use this time to breathe consciously and supply your body with oxygen. You can feel the sun on your skin and just enjoy it. Again, just start and try it out. You can start with a few minutes by simply walking around the block in the evening. If you are on holiday and have more time - or on weekends - you can take a longer walk or even a short hike. A walk on the beach or in the nearby woods is a great way to meditate while walking. You may also have a small lake, pond or stream in your area. Everything is possible and everything has a calming, relaxing effect on body, soul and spirit.

What you should keep in mind

Walk slowly and carefully. You have time. You want to meditate and relax, you don't have to achieve a goal. You now have an appointment with yourself. If it helps you to clarify your thoughts and clear your head, you can imagine your sequence of steps like a mantra: right-left-right-left or you can count your steps. You can also connect your breath with the steps: inhale - right foot, exhale - left foot.

If it's possible, avoid busy streets, choose quiet secondary streets, maybe you'll be lucky to have a park nearby. Also it is always good to take a bottle of water with you. It may be that you are so relaxed and that it does you so much good that you stay longer than planned. If you have more time, for example on weekends, pack a small backpack. Take enough to drink with you, maybe some fruit and a few nuts or something similar. Don't forget your rain jacket or sun hat and then just go. Let your intuition guide you and surprise you where you arrive.

Painting - meditation - Painting is a great way of relaxing and calming down. Maybe you just want to and have time to try it out? Then you can start right away... I have inserted a Mandala (https://www.free-mandalas.net) here for you, so that you can simply test it for yourself. Print out one or all three mandalas, get colorful pens, find a place to paint, sit down relaxed, take a few deep breaths and then let go of all thoughts of your daily life, stress and worries and sink completely into painting the mandala. I wish you a lot of joy with it. http://www.free-mandalas.net you will find many different mandalas to colour in, like for example this one:

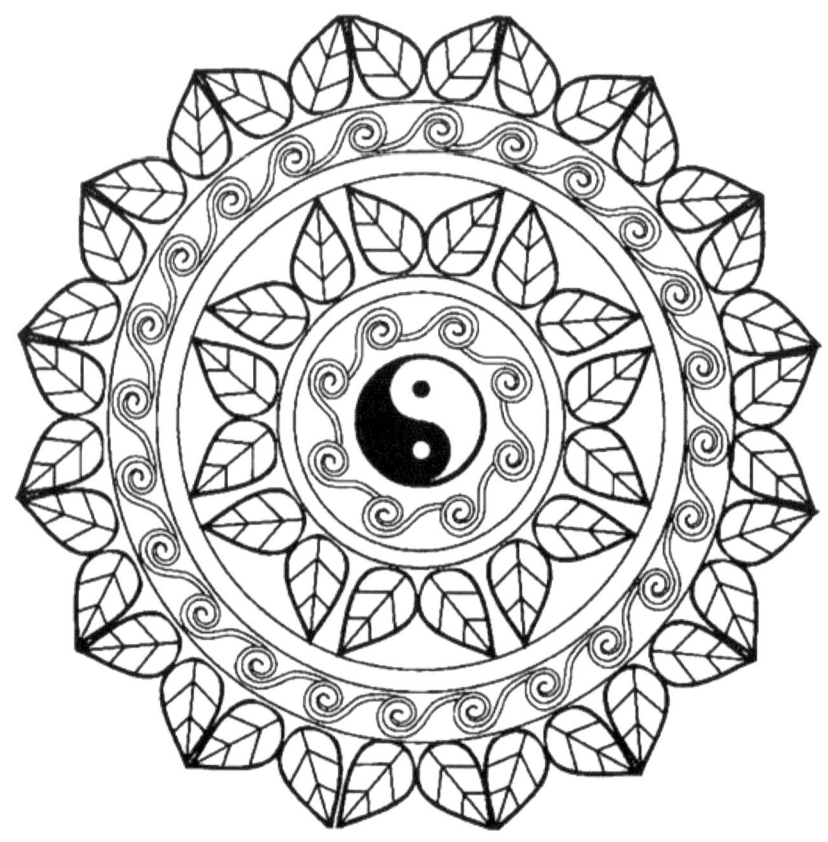

Another way to relax while painting and let your creativity come to light is medial painting. You need a piece of paper and paint and you can start. Everything ready? Then take a few deep breaths again, leave the daily routine behind you and start painting, let your intuition guide you, stop thinking. You will be amazed at what you find on paper. And believe me, YOU can also paint. If you feel like finding out more about this kind of relaxation, just come to my webinar "Mediales Malen", which takes place once a month. You can find current dates on my website.

Meditation in nature - If you enjoy spending time in nature, you can meditate wonderfully here as well. In my opinion this is something very special. For example, you can choose a beautiful old tree, get in touch with it, embrace it, and sit down on the ground to the roots of the tree. What do you feel? Which pictures come to you? Everything may be, let yourself in for it. Do breathing exercises and listen to the many sounds of nature. Or you can try the following: Imagine you are a tree, feel how your roots grow deep into the earth, feel the trunk, feel how the branches stretch into the sky, towards the sun, feel what it is like when the wind blows through the crown of the tree. At the end you take a few deep breaths again, extend and stretch yourself and come back to the daily consciousness.

At the end of your tree meditation it would be nice if you could thank your tree. Also in the mountains there are many places that invite you to stay and where you can do a meditation. Just sit down, let your gaze wander, let your thoughts wander, feel yourself. Other beautiful places for a meditation in nature can be a brook, a lake, the sea, a meadow, a forest clearing.

Just try out different places

Meditation in the Shower - Believe it or not, the shower is an excellent place to meditate. You are relaxed, the hot water helps you to feel purified and refreshed, and it is usually a quiet and calming room. And I'm sure you've meditated in the shower quite often without being aware of it. Read on to learn more about meditating in the shower.

Why the shower is a good place for your meditation - There are many different places where you can meditate, from sitting on your terrace to your bedroom with the door closed. The most important thing is that you choose a place which is quiet and peaceful and where you are not distracted and/or disturbed. This can be difficult when there are others at home who may knock on the door, come outside or enter your room looking for something. A better option is the shower. In most cases this time is just for you and there are far fewer distractions. The calm of the shower is the first reason why it is a good place to meditate. The combination of heat and steam coupled with the soothing sound of the water is another reason why it is the perfect place to meditate. Even before the actual meditation exercise, you may have noticed that you are more relaxed in the shower and always have the best ideas. There is a reason for this. To start showering meditation, you need to find something to concentrate on. As a beginner it may not be so easy to turn on the shower and relax the mind. Some people have so much on their mind that it is a bit more difficult. Find something in the shower to concentrate on. All you should do is focus on one thing, and that's it. This can be a thought, a mantra or an object you see. Some people just concentrate on the tap and watch the water come out while others try a mantra in the shower.

Use water to your advantage - Among the reasons why the shower is the perfect place for meditation is because you can use the water for meditation as well. The look, sound and soothing feeling of warm water on your skin can help you get rid of negative thoughts and focus on relaxation. If you have problems letting go of your thoughts and entering a meditative state, open your eyes and watch as the water flows out of the tap. Just stare it, listen to its flow and feel it on your skin. You can also imagine how the water washes away everything, negative thoughts, restlessness, sad feelings, lack of self-worth, etc... See how the water drains off and takes all that with it. Feel for yourself how you feel now. Much better already, isn't it? Meditating in the bathtub works similarly well. Many people can relax and let go even better there than in the shower. Just try it out.

Prayer as meditation - There isn't really much to write here. Every prayer can also be meditation. Turn every prayer into a little ritual for yourself, take time for your prayers. Whether you say the "Our Father" the rosary or a prayer with your own words is up to you. You can light a candle, use a prayer chain or a mala for help and then just start. Be sure, all prayers are heard.

Meditation for Insomnia - There are many ways meditation can help you, but one of the most important is to help you sleep better at night. If you regularly suffer from insomnia, it is advisable to help yourself in a more natural way instead of relying (only) on sleeping pills. The following information can help you to find a better and deeper sleep through meditation.

Why meditation works so well for insomnia - The reason why you should consider beginning meditating on your insomnia is this: it helps you relax your mind, stop the thought carousel. It is all too often that we have problems with falling asleep or sleeping through, not because we are not tired, but because we cannot get our head to stop thinking. Maybe you also have experienced this: You have had a hard day behind you, you are tired of falling down and just want to sleep, you go to bed and instead of sinking into your well-deserved sleep, the head carousel starts, you think of everything you said, did or did not do or said during the day. Small things suddenly become huge, you try to plan the morning and worry about dozens of other things, turn from one side to the other and can't find sleep. Here meditation and a few other little things can offer you valuable support. So if you meditate regularly in the evening before going to bed, body, mind and soul will be relaxed and in harmony. All the things that put you under stress every day will simply be washed away. With time it will be easier and easier for you to reach this soothing, relaxed place. This will not only help you to fall asleep, but also to sleep through and wake up fresh and rested the next morning.

Essential oils can promote good sleep - There are several essential oils that you can include in your meditation practice if you have sleep disorders:

  - Bergamot
  - Clary sage
  - Roman chamomile
  - Lavender
  - Ylang Ylang
  - Chamomile
  - Sandalwood
  - Basil

The best thing to do is to get some small samples of the aromatic oils. Fragrances are something very individual and you should feel really comfortable with your oil. You will have to try out which form of meditation helps you sleep better. Maybe it will help to leave out the TV in the evening and go for a walk instead, followed by a nice, relaxing shower. That would be a good start. Then you could either listen to a guided meditation or do one of the other meditations you have already learned. I wish you a restful sleep.

Zen Meditation - If you've ever seen someone sitting with his legs crossed and his eyes closed, he's most likely practicing Zen meditation. This is a kind of sitting meditation, similar to what Buddha did. You sit still and concentrate on your surroundings instead of your thoughts. You simply connect with your mind to clear it, concentrate on your breathing and not say a word. It is a silent meditation in which you gradually dive deeper and deeper into your subconscious to gain clarity and try to come into peace with yourself.

The Ten Steps of Zen

- – Let go of comparison.
- – Let go of competition
- – Let go of reviews
- – Let go of the trouble
- – Let go of the regret
- – Let go of your worries
- – Let go of recriminations.
- – Let go of the guilt
- – Let go of fear
- – Laugh at least once a day

That sounds simple and difficult at the same time, with Zen meditation you learn **mindfulness**. It's not about searching anymore, it's about finding. We are all constantly in search of love, recognition, wealth, money... And the more we search, the less we see what is there, in the here and now, in the moment. With this kind of meditation you take a step back, so to speak, direct your gaze towards yourself, come to your senses, then go on relaxed and with mindfulness. You give up your expectations and that is a big step towards more contentment and happiness. You can practice these ten steps every day, quite simply in your everyday life. Zen meditation is one of the most difficult types of meditation because you rely solely on your ability to be calm and try not to concentrate on anything. It definitely needs practice, so don't give up if you find it difficult the first time. As long as you have chosen the right time and place to sit in silence, you can get the hang of it.

Essential oils and meditation

When you start meditating, you will find that there are several ways to help you relax and come to rest. Through your sense of smell you can even get into relaxation very well and essential oils will help you. Let's have a look at a few possibilities: First you choose your favorite fragrance or mixture of fragrances. Then pour a few drops of it into a spray bottle filled with water. Shake well and then spray. The result is a very fine mist of scent that envelops you during meditation. You can also use an aroma lamp, where the water is mixed with a few drops of oil and a tea light is lit in the teapot underneath. Which can also be very pleasant: Mix a few drops of your preferred oil with a carrier oil such as jojoba or almond oil. Then rub one or two drops of this mixture onto your forehead in the area of the third eye. But beware: Please test beforehand whether you tolerate the oil well and do not react allergically. Alternatively, you can add a drop of essential oil to your T-shirt and inhale the fragrance well.

The best essential oils for meditation: The oils I present here will help you to focus, relax, concentrate and reduce your stress level. Try using only one at a time, or mix them to create your own relaxing fragrance blends. The point is: less is more. Here is a good list of essential oils to consider for meditation:

Cedar wood - really helps you not to think about anything and to concentrate more clearly during meditation.

Incense - is often used for meditation because it can help you to connect with your mind, it increases your vibration.

Sandalwood - Use sandalwood during meditation if you want to heal emotional or spiritual wounds.

Rose - Rose is an essential oil for love, even if you love yourself and learn to build a deeper connection to yourself.

Neroli - is a strong fragrance with which you allow yourself to accept yourself and face your fears. For your own fragrance blends, it may be useful to look at your themes and then make a blend. Let yourself be guided by your feelings.

Conclusion

This is where our journey through the world of meditation ends. I hope you have benefited from the different exercises and forms of meditation. Maybe you are already a meditation fan? I wish it for you. Please don't forget, meditation is a journey and as with any journey you need some patience and time. Don't give up on the first difficulties, start slowly and stick with it. Everybody can meditate, YOU too. You can download a guided morning meditation from me here as a special thank you, I wish you much joy.

bit.ly/morgen-meditation

CONTACT

Sandra Rauchenecker

E-Mail: kundenservice@sandra-rauchenecker.com
Internet: www.sandra-rauchenecker.com

Copyright and License Terms
The work, including all parts, is protected by copyright. This applies in particular to electronic or other reproduction, translation, distribution and making publicly available!

General information
The author has acted to the best of his knowledge and belief in the preparation of this book. Nevertheless, he does not guarantee the completeness, accuracy and practicability of the information presented in this book. Furthermore, no guarantees are given with regard to the profits to be achieved. Each reader is responsible for the use and implementation of the information presented in this

book. No liability is accepted for errors and the resulting consequences. All company names and product names mentioned in this book are trademarks or registered trademarks of their respective owners.

My recommendations for you

Meditationskissen   **https://amzn.to/2LCBpAW**

Meditationsbank   **https://amzn.to/2LCvMTc**

Primavera Airspray   **https://amzn.to/2FS9Akt**

Aromalampe mit Teelicht   https://amzn.to/2WSpiFY

Duftmischung Entspannung

Malen und entspannen: Meditation

Mandalas Zur Meditation: Ein Malbuch für Erwachsene

Mandalas Zum Malen und Entspannen: Punkt-zu-Punkt Meditation

 die passenden Stifte

About the author

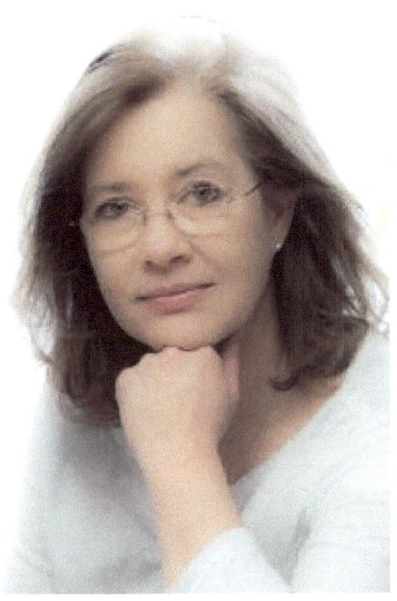

Sandra Rauchenecker was born in Munich in 1967, is happily married, has three grown-up children and in the meantime also her first grandchild. "Angels have always been around me - even though I wasn't always aware of it - they helped and are helping me and my family. Just as angels want to help everyone. My life is like that of everyone else, sometimes good, sometimes not so good. Faith in God and his angels has always been comfort and help." Often it is the difficult situations, the storms in our lives, where no stone remains on the other, that make us grow. We do not know how strong we are until we have lived through it and survived. Sometimes we rise from the ashes like phoenixes. Sandra herself has experienced this in many situations of her life. With her optimism and her big heart, she helps in every situation in life and gives everyone courage and strength again to accept their own way and to move on. Her personal life path has taught her a lot so far, her passion for healing has been ignited and strengthened again and again. For many years she has been dealing with all facets of healing and the angelic world. Out of her love for angels she created her first Guardian Angel Card Set in 2017. Since 2017 Sandra regularly participates in physical and healing circles and since recently she also leads her own healing circle. The connection to the spiritual world has let her recognize things, made her see and feel and she would like to pass that on. Sandra accompanies people on their way and supports them to see the light at the end of the tunnel and to let love and joy into their lives again. Also the stimulation of the self-healing powers, the healthy on all levels of being, is a matter close to her heart.

MY TRAININGS

Nurse,
Reiki up to Master's degree,
Relaxation pedagogy,
Aroma oil and gemstone therapy,
Angel Light Healing,
Angel medium,
Energy medicine,
Pendulum course,
Golden energy healing,
Distance learning Akasha Chronicle,
Media distance learning,
Trance healing,
Distance learning shamanic healing methods,
Hospice companion.